Christ, Cancer

~N~

Chemo

Christ, Cancer

~N~

Chemo

Sabino ~N~ Beatrice

Library of Congress Control Number:		2012902143
ISBN:	Hardcover	978-1-4691-6225-6
	Softcover	978-1-4691-6224-9
	Ebook	978-1-4691-6226-3

All Bible quotations used in this book were taken from the King James Version 1611.

This book was printed in the United States of America.

To order additional copies of this book, contact:
Xlibris Corporation
1-888-795-4274
www.Xlibris.com
Orders@Xlibris.com
109336

Contents

For God hath not given us the spirit of fear; but of power, and of love, and of a sound mind.

2 Timothy 1:7

Prologue

There was darkness all around me with very little light still left to see. So I walked slowly. Carefully. Seeing a rather tall figure approaching me, I slowed down my pace. When the ominous-looking figure reached me, it began fighting with me. I soon realized it was the devil himself. Not *a* devil, but *the* devil. He fought fiercely, but so did I. Blow for blow, kick for kick the fight went on. I was terrified as I fought on. He was horrific up close. Indescribable hatred showed up close on his face, not just for me but for all of mankind. The fight carried on for quite a while. At long last we backed away from each other. It was a draw. Suddenly I woke up. It had been another nightmare. Being a Christian, I felt very disappointed that I had not been able to win the fight even if it was just a dream. After all, being a born-again believer, don't I have the Holy Ghost residing in me as promised in the book of Ephesians chapter 1, verse 13 of the Holy Bible? And the Bible also says in 1 John 4:4 that greater is he that is in you than he that is in the world. But in the dream I just had, how come I lost the fight to the devil? It didn't make any sense to me at that time. In reality, it would take me a full year of my life for me to really understand the full meaning of that dream. I'll confess that I do believe in dreams to some extent. But I sure don't go around setting myself to live by them. After all, did not the Lord give ample warning to the wise men against Herod in a dream (Matthew 2:12)? And Joseph also in a dream was warned not to leave Mary, when she was found to be with child (Matthew 1:20). And what about the warning that reached Pontius Pilate's wife through a dream just before the crucifixion of our Lord Jesus? In dreams, God also spoke to King Solomon, the prophet Daniel, King Nebuchadnezzar, Joseph in Egypt, and many others. I didn't quite realize it yet, but this particular dream was a foreboding to me of one of the biggest physical and spiritual battles that I would ever go through in my life. The prince of darkness was fast approaching me, and I didn't even know it.

Chapter 1

A MYSTERIOUS ILLNESS

January 8, 2009—I arrived home in the evening after a hard day's work. I am a welder by trade. The company I work for is a maintenance company. So when there's no welding to be done, I do carpentry, concrete work, or even be a laborer. My job then was at a refinery in Corpus Christi, Texas. However, my wife and I are renting in Portland. It's just over the Harbor Bridge north of Corpus Christi; about three more miles and there's our home.

I got home that evening to find my wife cooking a fine supper. Her name is Beatrice, and she's been with two different school districts for a total of seventeen years. She's a bus driver and truly loves her job and the people she works with, especially all the little kiddos she carries in her bus with her during the week. I went into the kitchen where she was cooking and gave her a quick hug and a kiss. No sooner had I done that than I began feeling instantly sick in the stomach. Running to the restroom, I quickly threw up. My wife and I couldn't figure what had brought that on. I mean, I just had a really great day at work. There wasn't even any pain anywhere in my body. Sure, I had some unexplained weight loss, but overall I felt pretty good.

After the ugly episode in the restroom, I quickly showered. We then had a real nice supper. The rest of the evening went on by with no further incidents.

In the morning, we both got up pretty excited partly because it was Friday. We were both looking forward to spending a good weekend together. As strange as it sounds to a lot of people around us, we still very much enjoy spending as much time together as we could. I am not really possessive of my wife at all. In the past, I've let her go on and enjoy herself on trips with her friends to such places as San Antonio, Houston, and even Mexico. With our thirty-fifth wedding anniversary just a week away, I was happy as a lark. That is, until I suddenly started feeling sick all over again. It was about five twenty in the morning, and here I was throwing up all over again. And for no reason in the world too. Or so I thought.

Afterward, I washed up all over again. Getting dressed for work, I then joined Beatrice in the kitchen. Of course, she was very concerned about me. She suggested I go see our family doctor over in Sinton, which is about twenty-two miles away from Portland. We had just sold our place in Sinton and had just recently moved to Portland. I agreed with her to go in for a checkup. Except for feeling extremely bloated, I felt rather fine.

Calling in sick, I took off to see the doctor around 8:30 a.m. Since I had no prior appointment, he finally saw me about 10:30 a.m. The doctor pointed out that my spleen was very swollen, which accounted for my feeling bloated. As he continued to check me over, I noticed a certain look come over him, like he already knew what it could be but was uncertain about telling me. They did some blood work on me there and then. He sent me to the radiologist in Portland for an MRI on my stomach. These would be done Monday morning.

After the MRI Monday morning, I drove back to Sinton to see the doctor. He set me up for another MRI. This one would be done on my upper back. He had noticed a good-size lump on my upper side of my left shoulder blade. I always knew about it and had thought it was caused by an overworked pulled muscle. I began missing a lot of work. Days turned into weeks, and still we didn't have a clue as to what could be ailing me.

February 4—At my sister's bidding, my Beatrice took me to the Shoreline Sphon Hospital in Corpus Christi. My sister, Rita, who is a nurse there, insisted that by my looks alone I needed to go in. About this time, considerable weight loss could be seen on me. According to the medical staff every single lymph node in my body was swollen and painful too. After several hours in the hospital, I was sent home. We were pretty well shaken by the news the lady doctor had given us there. In a very sweet and professional manner, she had told us that she had a strong suspicion that cancer was at the bottom of our problem.

February 13—This time we found ourselves at the Sphon South Hospital in Corpus Christi. There we were informed that they would proceed to take out the most severe looking lymph node I had. That one turned out to be the one I had on my upper left-hand side on my groin area. The road of life had just begun to get a little rough for me now.

Chapter 2

MORE BAD NEWS

February 19—My wife and I were having supper one evening when our oncologist called us on our cell. Answering the cell, she was the first one to receive the terrible news. Just seeing her expression, I could tell she was clearly upset by what she'd just heard. Upon relating the news to me, I just reclined back in my chair. Calmly I related to her how in the past the Lord had blessed us both with a very good and happy marriage of thirty-five years already, and that he had allowed us to see all three of our children grow up, and that he had even blessed us with two grandchildren. I explained to her how we had both been saved a long time already and that, personally speaking, I was ready to go be with the Lord if that be his will. I continued that I had heard and read so much about what heaven must be like. I was almost positive I was ready to go right then and there. So knowing that I was saved and going to heaven, I believed I had every right to be cheerful and happy. After all, I didn't exactly choose this disease upon me on purpose. Besides, whining, crying, and complaining about it wasn't going to help my circumstances any or improve my present situation, right? If you ask me, I was pretty well excited about the whole thing. I thought it was great. But the thought of going through the door of death kind of had me a little concerned. I didn't want to suffer too much. But if that was the only way to get there, so be it. I did have one big regret about the whole thing though. And that was that I felt real sorry for my loved ones I was leaving behind.

The great attitude I possessed was possible because I was a born-again believer. And it was the indwelling of the Holy Spirit that was giving me all my comfort and confidence in the Lord now. It gave me the necessary courage to help pick up my wife's spirit and to be a great encouragement to her during the whole year that I was stricken with this dreadful disease. I knew I hadn't been living for him the way I should. My style of living was okay, but I knew I could've done a lot better. At this point in my illness, this scripture came to my attention: "It is good that I have been afflicted; that I might learn thy statutes" (Psalm 119:71).

Some days later, the oncologist removed some bone marrow from my lower back. For this procedure, I had to lie down on my side in a fetal position. The minor operation was painful enough and felt like someone was hammering on my lower back. Afterward, some patients in there said that it was a rather painless procedure and that it really depended on the oncologist performing it at the time.

Right after the bone marrow removal, the oncologist showed me a small jar with a lid on it. It was about an inch in diameter and about one and a half inches tall. It was also full of my spinal fluid. And floating around inside was a small sliver of bone about an inch or so in length that had also been cut out of me. I don't know how in the world they had extracted that out of me without paralyzing me, but there it was.

Our oncologist explained to us that this particular medical test would determine if the cancer I possessed had gone into my skeletal system. He said that four of the major cancers are mesothelioma, melanoma, leukemia, and lymphoma. Under lymphoma, which I just happened to have, there are forty categories. These are divided into two separate groups called Hodgkin's and non-Hodgkin's. I was in the non-Hodgkin's group. And the particular non-Hodgkin's cancer I had was called stage 4 mantel cell lymphoma. On a stage level of 1 through 4, 1 being the lowest and 4 being the highest and most dangerous, I had reached stage 4. Everyone with a stage 4 lymphoma must take a spinal tap to determine if that cancer has gone into their bones. This test later showed us that I had mantel cell lymphoma throughout my skeletal system.

March 17—Because I was missing so much work, my employer laid me off on March 10. I had just missed a whole week of work at that time. But due to the fact that more medical work needed to be done on me, I went ahead and requested a few more days off. They told me not to worry about coming back to work. I didn't understand why. So when I inquired about it, they informed me that I'd been laid off a week back. As we've both done in the past, my wife and I silently thanked the Lord. We knew that everything was going according to his plan. Sometime later we drove to the refinery to pick up my personal belongings. Two of my friends drove out of the plant to bring them to me. Both are God-fearing men and very hardworking. They gave me my things and said their good-byes. They then each gave me a big hug and placed well over $200 in my hand. According to what they told me, every man in our crew had pitched in to give us this financial blessing. Later on they repeated this love offering for us again with $300. As sure as I sit here writing out this personal testimony, I know that God will one day bless each and every one of those men for their act of kindness.

All this didn't change my attitude about life or worry me in the least. I continued to praise his mighty name and to trust in him. Without the Lord Jesus in my heart, I know I would've gone mentally to pieces long ago. I was totally amazed at his presence and the way he was working in my life now that I was so ill. My personal outlook on life had become so good that it effected a lot of people around me. Some were blessed by it while others took offense at it. The latter group said that by treating it so lightly and joking about it, I was surely inviting more disaster into my life. A few even thought I had finally gone off the deep end. To all this, I could only reply with "My God is so great that he laughs at cancer."

Chapter 3

I SEE A DEAD MAN WALKING

About a week before I started on chemotherapy, a PowerPort was surgically embedded just under my skin. It was placed on my upper right-hand side of my chest. Through this PowerPort, I was to receive all my chemo and most of my medication. It was a small gadget, about an inch in thickness and approximately a square inch all the way around. A small hose was attached to the PowerPort while the loose end that was left was inserted into one of the main arteries going into my heart.

Whenever I went into the hospital for chemo, a regular-size needle with a short section of surgical tubing attached to it was inserted into my PowerPort. This surgical tubing was approximately four inches long. To it were attached several more sections of tubing of various lengths that had plastic Y's attached to the ends. This would allow more tubing to be added as needed. To the ends of all these were attached clear plastic bags full of chemo or other types of medication. Sometimes, I would have as many as six bags feeding me all types of fluids and medication. These bags would all be suspended from the top of a tall metal stand with small rubber wheels underneath. Believe me, sleeping with a bunch of hoses attached to one's body is no picnic. And these would remain attached to me for the duration of each chemo treatment. All that was happening to me and that I was going through was new to me. I had never been through something like this in my life. But I steadily continued with my faith in God and took it all in stride. One day at a time.

Before any of the chemo treatments began, we visited my mom and dad, who live in Sinton. My older brother whose wife passed away many years ago also lives there. My wife and I gave them the bad news of my recent medical condition. My dad took it bravely enough, but my mom was somewhat broken up about it. After our visit, we all stood outside saying our good-byes. We were all gathered at the end of their driveway when our aunt and uncle drove up for a visit. Since we were already leaving, I quickly broke the bad news about me to them too. My uncle just sadly shook his head and told us how sorry he was to hear that. My aunt, on the other hand, took one good, long look at me. We expected some kind of word of encouragement. Instead, what we heard her say came as a complete shock to us. She said my cousin had been found with an advanced cancer of some type just like me and that he hadn't made it. In fact, I probably wouldn't live past six months.

Although my uncle looked embarrassed by what she said, he didn't say a single word to her. For that matter, neither did anyone else. Including me. Hearing all this did get me to thinking though. How terrible must be the faith and the hope of those that are eternally lost. Their hope is easily crushed when faced with insurmountable odds. And their faith too is easily vanquished, seeing it hasn't been anchored on Christ Jesus.

Chapter 4

THE WONDERFUL WORLD OF CHEMO

At first, I thought I was going to be receiving my chemotherapy there at the clinic, which was only about a block away from the main hospital on Shoreline. On several occasions, I had observed other cancer patients receiving their chemo while sitting down on what resembled real nice-looking recliners. After, anywhere from two to three hours, they were done with the chemo and allowed to go home. That is, until the following day, week, or month when it would be time for their next treatment. A friend of ours was doing her chemo in San Angelo. Hers was once a month, which sounded okay to me. But in November, they gave her a week off from her treatments because of the holidays. Pretty cool, I thought. Maybe I would end up getting about the same chemo treatments as her. Boy, was I ever wrong.

I'll never forget my first experience with chemo. For my first treatment, we were told to be there Monday by six am and by 8:00 a.m., I had been admitted. Immediately the hospital staff worked on getting me hooked up onto my PowerPort. I wasn't released from the hospital until late Friday afternoon. I had been hooked up for five days in a row for a total of approximately 105 hours. My dreams of kicking back and relaxing on a recliner while receiving chemo for a couple of hours were totally dashed to pieces.

Originally, our oncologist had said that I would be receiving chemo every three weeks. At the end of our first week of treatment, he informed us that it had been changed to every two weeks now. I didn't respond to any of this as they wheeled me out in a wheelchair. I was devastated. I felt totally wasted by the chemo. As our oncologist had explained earlier, chemo, although a powerful, effective medicine for fighting cancer, is nothing short of pure poison—a very dangerous but reliable poison that is pumped into one's system. It not only destroys off dangerous cancer cell but kills off one's immune system. Not to mention making that person sick as a dog.

And that's exactly how I felt after receiving my little dose of chemo. I knew a person was to feel kind of ill afterward. But besides feeling ill, it seemed like anything that could go wrong or happen to me did. I don't know why it did. Maybe it was the age factor involved. After all, I wasn't a teenager anymore. I was fifty-six years old now. For the duration of my chemo sessions, I managed to experience just about every bad side effect there was to a chemo treatment. I didn't go through all of them at once, thank goodness. However, I always did have several plaguing me at any one time.

To begin with, my spleen was now completely swollen all across my stomach. It made me feel so bloated with just about anything I would eat. My bones in my body would ache terribly sometimes, especially those in my legs. Week after week didn't go by that I did not feel nauseated. Finding myself throwing up in a restroom became a routine thing for me. All my life I have enjoyed eating all types of hot peppers and spicy foods. Now I couldn't do it any longer. The inside of my mouth had become extremely sensitive. Anything even slightly spicy would make it feel like the inside of my mouth was burning.

Even brushing my teeth became a very painful experience for me because of the toothpaste. Rinsing my mouth with any kind of mouthwash solution was unbearable. A very small meal that was only a bit spicy would leave the top part of my head and backside completely drenched in cold sweat. Then came the night sweats. This too came about because of the cancer.

Before long, I began experiencing shortness of breath. Going at a fast walk from the front of our house to the backyard would leave me all tuckered out and breathing hard. Finding myself with plenty of time on my hands, I decided to clean out the garage one day. However, after working for about twenty or twenty-five minutes, I became so sick with exhaustion that I almost had to crawl back into the house. It took me that day and the greater part of the next to completely get over it. Through medical tests done on me, I found out later on that my lungs had been damaged by the chemo. When I stumbled half dazed into the house that day, I went straight to our bedroom and threw myself onto the bed. As I lay there gagging and coughing, a strange thought came to my mind. Just one year ago, I had been training myself for the Beach to Bay Run. Although the team had broken up and we hadn't done the run, I had still been able to do a pretty decent five-mile practice run.

Forgetfulness was another side effect. Concentrating and remembering things became very difficult. Simple elementary arithmetic was more than a chore for me. Sitting one day at our kitchen table, I tried to add up a small list of two-digit numbers. Hard as I tried, it became almost an impossible task. I added them over and over again. Several times. But after each try, I would come up with a different total. I finally gave up in total frustration. It didn't take long before my mistakes began to show up at the bank, at grocery stores, while paying our rent, and in other places. As if that wasn't bad enough, whenever I get up from a sitting or lying position, I would hear a real loud pounding noise in my ears. Then a wave of dizziness would overtake me. Finally, after easing off me, the whole thing would pass after four to five minutes. From the time I first became ill to well over a year later, I had a roaring type of noise going on constantly inside my head. Day and night it went on. It would never go away. It resembled the type of noise a jet airliner makes when slowly passing overhead. Not loud enough, yet enough that it would seem that a regular person might easily go nuts from hearing it. Thank God that he helped me to endure it so that in time I was able to learn to live with it. Most nights, in order that I might fall asleep, I would rig me up a radio with earphones. This helped a lot in drowning out the noise. Plus, it was also nice in that it helped me to fall asleep while listening to good music.

Chapter 5

MORE SIDE EFFECTS

Soon after the chemo sessions began, I developed a real bad case of skin dryness. It was all over my arms, legs, and other parts of my body. My eyes went bad too. I would see blurry sometimes, and my eyes would be very itchy constantly. In time I was able to obtain eye medication from our doctors in Sinton, Corpus Christi, and San Antonio. These itchy-blurry spells would come upon me as they pleased. I was never able to figure them out. No matter how much medication I poured into my eyes, the symptoms always managed to return.

Also, my limbs would twitch and jerk crazily all over the place every night. Never during the day. This would only take place in the evenings when I went to bed to sleep. This particular side effect would work on one arm. Other times both arms. Sometimes one leg, while other nights it would hit both. It even attacked my back and also my head. For example, I'd be lying comfortably in bed when all of a sudden my head would jerk violently sideways as far as it could possibly go. I felt like what little girl in the movie *The Exorcist* must've felt. These attacks would hit me every two to three minutes and would last for as long as it took me to fall asleep. I still remember dreading to go to sleep at night. I recall one evening when a nurse walked in on me in the middle of the night to find me with my legs kicking all over the place. She was shocked and thought I was having an epilepsy attack.

Insomnia came into my life immediately after my chemo began. To a cancer victim, rest is very important in every sense of the word. With insomnia in the picture now, things were sure going to get interesting for me. I passed the nights by reading or watching sci-fi and old classics on the cable channel. Sleep just eluded me. If I did fall asleep, it'd be around four or five in the morning. And then I'd be awake again by seven or seven thirty in the morning. I hated it, being awake at night. Our oncologist prescribed diazepam, zolpidem, and Valium as the days slowly rolled by. But my nights still continued to be sleepless and miserable on the outside. But on the inside, my faith and hope in the Lord remained high.

One thing that really bugged me to death was the ugly, nasty metallic taste I had acquired inside my mouth. Even most foods now held a certain disgusting smell that's hard to describe. I remember not being able to open certain cabinet doors in our kitchen because the smell of food inside them would gag me. Some sections of the grocery store were also avoided by me because the smell of foods there would also turn my stomach. Sometimes, we'd be blessed and be able to go out to eat in a restaurant. The trouble was that, hard as I tried, my appetite had now been cut in half. And most of the food I ate held no taste for me. I would say that I could find some sort of taste in about less than 5 percent of the meals I had. Everything I did manage to consume tasted much like paper with a tiny bit of food flavoring in it. The average American in the United States is used to eating well at home and even enjoying a nice meal at some fast-food place or good restaurant once a week. At least once a week, I dare say. Maybe even more. Food can become a terrible temptation, if you know what I mean. Just recall from the Holy Bible what it was that Satan used in order to tempt Eve—food.

As Beatrice and I walked along the beach one evening, I felt like it might just be a good idea to fill my pockets full of rocks in order to keep the wind from blowing me away. The way my pant legs were flapping around in the wind, they reminded me of sails on a sailboat. I did hold on to my wife though. People passing us by thought we looked very romantic by the comments they made. They really didn't know that I was holding on to her to keep from falling. Later on I resorted to using a cane to help steady me and for me to lean on while I caught my breath, especially when the waves of dizziness would suddenly hit me. I know I was very weak and that I looked terrible on the outside. But during the times when the side effects of chemo weren't torturing me, my wife would take me out for walks. She said that it was a good exercise for me. As she and I walked, I thought of the numerous outings she and I had during our life together when our children were growing up. And then we'd only have a handful of vacations together. But they had been very memorable. Now to me, a simple walk along the beach had become a joyous occasion. Little did Adam and Eve know what type of suffering and heartache they were to bring upon mankind when they disobeyed God in the Garden of Eden.

Our best and only daughter, April, who is a teacher in a private school at the Heritage Baptist Church in Lawrence, Kansas, came over to spend the summer with us. Every year she comes home to visit us but only for about two weeks. But Brother Hanks, who is the pastor there, suggested to her that she come home for the whole summer to help take care of me. Not only was he thoughtful enough to do that, but he even allowed her to come a whole month before school let out. So we ended up greeting her at the Corpus Christi airport in the month of May.

April has always been a great blessing to us. Now she had volunteered her personal time to help take care of me while my wife continued to work. By this time, I was being driven around like an invalid. My mental capacities were shod. My memory lapses came and went. I was completely unreliable. Whenever my health permitted, I would do my best to enjoy life to the fullest with good fellowship with my loved ones.

After each and every chemo treatment I received, my white blood cell count would go down to zero, which meant I had absolutely no immune system to combat anything contagious I might contract from the outside world. To counteract this predicament, they would inject me with Neupogen, a medication that helped boost up my white blood cell count. I received these types of injections twice a week, sometimes three times. Toward the end of my ordeal, I would be getting them morning and night, one day after another. As if all this wasn't bad enough, the devil was about to throw another monkey wrench into the works again.

May 16—It being a beautiful Saturday afternoon and all, we all decided to go biking. Beatrice and April loaded up all three bikes in the back of our pickup and drove over to the water's edge. Portland has a real neat-looking bike trail. Part of it overlooks the Corpus Christi Bay. Beyond the water you can see the gigantic Harbor Bridge with a large part of the city standing out in the background. The skyscrapers along with the famous ship the *Lexington* and other large water vessels in the ship channel give it a most magnificent view. Our biking was great. Afterward, they loaded the bikes back up in our truck and headed back home. None of us knew then that I wouldn't be riding another bike for the rest of the year.

Chapter 6

WELCOME TO ICU

After our biking, we headed back home. While Beatrice and April prepared an afternoon snack, I sat out in the front porch to rest. I was amazed. I had just enjoyed a great bike ride with my little family, and it made me feel good inside. While I was still enjoying my emotional high, the devil pulled out the rug from under my feet.

Suddenly I began getting chills. Going inside the house, I lay down on our bed, shaking the whole time. My wife called the hospital and quickly explained my condition along with my cancer situation. They advised her to take me in, and within minutes, I was admitted into the hospital and straight into ICU. My fever was recorded at 105.9. Accompanying the fever was an excruciating headache that was making me feel like my skull was splitting in half. My brain felt like it was on fire.

My immediate family came into ICU to see me. Our church pastor, faithful as ever, showed up to pray for me. I guess they all thought I was a real goner. My pain was so intense in my whole body that I refused to speak to anyone in the room. I just lay there holding my head in my hands. I silently prayed that he would help me to endure the pain and to just shine for him regardless of how bad I felt.

Cancer and chemo can wreck havoc in one's life. One day you feel like you can do things almost like a normal person, and the next thing you know you feel like you're dying. One day you enjoy a nice, leisurely walk or even a bike ride, but the next day someone has to help you get around inside your own house.

I had lost so much weight that I now looked like a human skeleton. My natural color was now gone. My appearance was very pale with a pasty yellowish color. The hair on my head, arms, legs, even my eyebrows was completely gone now. Going through long, intense chemo treatments was really taking its toll on me. Nothing pleases the devil more than to come in and destroy one's health as he did to Job as mentioned in the Bible in the book of Job chapter 2, verse 7. He loves nothing better than to wreck people's marriages, their finances, testimony, and other things that are important to us. If he can influence a person to give up on God and life itself, he can drive that person to commit suicide.

All over the Bible, God commands us to be courageous and be good soldiers of the cross. Well, a real soldier is supposed to be tough and able to endure hardship. And I knew I was a soldier of the cross. So having the Lord Jesus dwelling in my heart had taken away all fear of dying. But just because I wasn't afraid to die did not mean I was just going to keel over and give up the ghost that easily. If that was what the devil thought, he had another thing coming. The Lord had blessed me with wisdom, good doctors, a great hospital staff to attend to me, plus the fervent prayers of many of his saints. So all this meant that I was going to go down fighting. I decided right then and there that all my suffering was nothing. After all, Jesus went through a lot more for us on the cross on Calvary, did he not?

I requested several ice packs from the nurses. They managed to bring them over to me immediately. The nurses asked me what I planned to do with so much ice. I quickly explained to them, and they agreed that it would help me. I repeated this procedure hour after hour until the fever finally broke.

The fever did continue but not as high as before. It would come back on and off. Up one moment and down the next. It finally leveled off at ninety-nine degrees. I was trembling and exhausted and soaking wet from melted ice, but with God's help, I had managed to pull through. My headaches continued on. They went on for days, then weeks. Different medications were tried on me, but nothing seemed to help. Morphine injections seemed to control them somewhat, but even then, it was only temporarily. Many medical tests were done on me to determine the cause of my headache, including a brain scan. Nothing could be found. Fearing meningitis, the doctors ordered a spinal tap. It also came out negative. In the months to follow, I would be taking a whole assortment of painkillers for this newest ailment that was now plaguing me. Not to mention all the medication I was already receiving in the hospital and at home. I had become a literal walking medicine cabinet. After being in ICU for seven whole days, I was released from the hospital. Just before leaving, the doctors advised me to go straight home, make sure I took all my medication, and be sure I got plenty of rest. "Phew, what a terrific spiritual and physical battle I have just gone through," I thought. But after seven days, I found myself back in the hospital for my fifth round of chemo.

June 8—My fifth round of chemo I received turned out to be my last one that I would take in Corpus Christi. Before I began receiving chemotherapy, our oncologist had informed us that I would be getting six chemo treatments in Corpus Christi. The seventh one, which would be a type of real harsh and very strong chemo, would be taken in the city of Houston, at MD Anderson Hospital. Besides the heavy-duty chemo, I would also be going through a bone marrow transplant. However, things had changed now. Our oncologist informed us that they were going to forgo the sixth treatment in Corpus Christi and go straight on to the seventh one in Houston. Reason being was that from their professional point of view, my body couldn't take it anymore. I had gone through some real bad side effects that are associated with chemo. Not some of them, but all of them. My body had retaliated and fought against the chemo the whole way to now. He said they couldn't understand why I kept reacting so badly to all my treatments. Frankly, he admitted he saw no way how my body would be able to withstand another round of chemo.

I had literally spent hundreds of hours hooked up while receiving bodily fluids, chemo, and various other medications. And now my body was just plain worn out and couldn't take any more. Ironically, I had celebrated my fifty-sixth birthday while going through my first chemo session. Imagine that. A real mystery with plenty of unanswered questions. At last a realistic and concrete answer finally seemed to surface. Perhaps the Lord was allowing the devil to deal out his very worst against me so that in the end he would eventually glorify himself by performing a miraculous healing on me.

Chapter 7

VACATIONING IN SAN ANTONIO

Our oncologist asked us if we wanted our last medical treatment to be at MD Anderson in Houston or at the Methodist Hospital in San Antonio. He said they were both very competent and professionally sound in all their medical accomplishments in the cancer field. Since they both sounded pretty good, we settled on going to the one in San Antonio. Upon hearing this, our nephew Robert and his wife, Marilu, invited us to stay with them. Robert is an AC tech in San Antonio while Marilu is a licensed vocational nurse at one of the San Antonio hospitals. She also served in the war in Iraq and is now an officer in the Army Reserve. Their little boy, Danny, is ten years old and is a crossroad guard in school. He is also an excellent karate student with a third-degree brown belt. Taking violin lessons, he hopes to one day be able to play "The Devil Went Down to Georgia" better than Charlie Daniels himself.

Staying at their place turned out to be an even greater blessing than we thought. You see, their home is located just about a mere twenty minutes away from the hospital we would be going to. We were going to be in San Antonio for over a month, so financially this was going to be a big help to us.

Our oncologist had instructed us to check in to the Methodist Hospital in about eight more weeks. The reason for this was that they wanted all the chemo to come out of my body so that they could run a CAT scan to see if I was in remission. Later, it proved that I was. But they were afraid that there might be some cancer cells still floating around inside my bones. So that's where the cell transplant would come into play. Of course, the real harsh chemo would also play a big part in that too.

July 30—I arrived in San Antonio with my wife and daughter. I looked half dead, like a bug that has been stepped on, but I arrived anyhow. I was a terrible sight, but I joked and laughed along with everyone else like I was normal or something.

Our nephew and his little family came out of their house to greet us. They have a fairly nice and big-enough house along with a good-size driveway. On the driveway stood an attractive RV with a spacious living quarters of six feet by twelve feet. With three bunk beds, kitchen table, shower, bathroom, and kitchen appliances, plus 3 people tramping around inside it, I just knew it was going to be an adventure living in it.

We unloaded our luggage and did our best to get ourselves settled in. The first night, we kept bumping into one another, stepping on one another's feet, hitting ourselves on our shinbones, and knocking stuff off the furniture. Beatrice slept on the bunk bed by the door at the front end of the little RV. On the back end were two more bunk beds, one on top of the other. April took the top one while I readily took the one at the bottom. During the night, I kept bumping my knees hard against the wall. Other times I would smash my head against the bottom of the top bunk, where April was sleeping. On a couple of occasions, she even stepped on me trying to get to her own bunk. A claustrophobic person wouldn't have lasted too long in there. They would've run out screaming the first night. Unbelievable as it sounds, we began to soon find the little RV quite cozy and very comfortable. On the days when the sun would seem like it was about to burn everything up outside, we would stay inside it, relaxing. We would look outside, and it would look like everything was getting roasted and toasted. On those days, we would just kick back and enjoy the nice AC. Looking outside through the window by my bunk bed, I could still see God's hand working in all that was happening to us.

Chapter 8

MANNA FROM GOD'S PEOPLE

It is interesting to note here that during the whole time that I was sick, there were people praying for us from the Corpus Christi area and surrounding towns. There were prayer warriors up in San Antonio, the state of Oklahoma, and even Kansas. Church pastors would show up at our doorstep and ask to come in and pray for us. I was always coming across people that would say they had me on their prayer list even though I had never even met them. People we didn't know would hold benefits to raise money for our financial needs. We received a great deal of help from the Catholic Church, Baptist Church, Methodists, and many others in the area. Organizations like the Salvation Army, Portland Municipal Foundation, and the Sinton Community Action Center really blessed us.

Ironically, we were unable to obtain help from the Texas Employment Commission. They insisted I wouldn't qualify for unemployment unless I went out there to look for work five times a week. This proved rather impossible for me since I was so ill most of the time and always under medication. Under this condition, no one would ever hire me.

So next, Beatrice sought help at the Human Resources in Sinton. At that time, we had $450 in the bank. Noticing this, the case worker there told my wife that we would never qualify because we had too much money sitting in the bank. My wife then explained to her that by the end of the month the rent would be due and that in itself would come to $650. So in the meantime, where was she supposed to keep all that money? And besides that, we still had to save up a lot more for the new car we were paying on. Hearing all this, the lady callously replied that we had to get rid of the car because we had no business owning a new vehicle while applying for food stamps. My wife just turned around and left the place and never went back.

During the summer of my illness, our little '97 Geo Metro spent an entire three-month period in the auto repair shop. Twice on the way home from the repair shop it broke down and had to be hauled back again. On three other separate occasions, it broke down also and was fixed up in another auto repair shop. But then again, what do you expect from a run-down twelve-year-old vehicle. It's still going though. Thank the Lord that during the whole time that our little car was in the shop receiving chemo of its own, we had the new car to carry us about, which was what Beatrice was using the whole time we were in San Antonio. I suppose it wouldn't have made a difference to tell all this to the lady at the Human Resources. Anyway, the whole time that major agencies were refusing us help, God was raining down manna from heaven to us through the people who love him.

God has truly demonstrated his power in all this. Sure my wife works for the Portland Independent School District and does housecleaning as a side job. But just the car payment and the medical insurance alone completely wipe her school check out. Yet through the miracle of the Lord's love for us, we have never failed to give our rent money or a car payment on time. The Lord has faithfully supplied all our needs. Truthfully the Bible says it all in the book Of Isaiah in chapter 59, verse 19, where it reads: "When the enemy shall come in like a flood, the Spirit of the Lord shall lift up a standard against him."

Chapter 9

TIME FOR A SPIRITUAL CHECKUP

My friend, if Satan is attacking you today in some area of your life, the worst thing you can do is to give up hope. Commit all your troubles to the Lord and lay them down at his feet. They are his problems, not yours. Our Lord Jesus came to die on the cross as a sacrifice for our sins. A supreme sacrifice that would ensure salvation for us if we trust and accept him as our savior. The first priority in your life right now is to call upon him to forgive you for all your sins and invite him into your heart. The Bible says in Ephesians 2:8 and Titus 3:5 that we will never be able to attain heaven by good works. This automatically rules out our religion. Long ago, our pastor from the old church used to tell us that religion would never make you into a Christian no more than living in a car garage would turn you into a car. John chapter 3 tells us that a very religious man was told by Jesus that he needed to be born again.

John 3:36 says that if you haven't been saved, you are condemned already. Not later or in the day of Judgment but right now. Not after your good deeds have been weighed against your bad deeds either, but already. After receiving the Lord Jesus as your personal savior, then and only then should you concentrate on getting the affairs of your health straightened out. You see, what will it profit you to receive God's miracle healing only to later die of old age or for whatever reason and find yourself in hell?

First take care of your spiritual priorities, and then after doing that, go back and get concerned about taking care of your personal health.

Remember, Satan has been around for thousands of years, and he is a master of deception and discouragement. He knows every single weakness you possess and will stop at nothing to disappoint you, discourage you, and finally, break you.

One hot summer day when I was at home feeling pretty low—that's a health concern, not a spiritual or emotional one. Anyhow, Beatrice came home to find me cheerfully plugging away at my guitar. She was looking a little perplexed, so I asked her what the matter was. She answered and said that some time in the morning, her friend had gotten in touch with her by cell phone. And according to her friend, I was suffering from cancer because I was allowing it in my life through unbelief in the power of healing. If I would just be willing to get up and drive over to their church and allow their pastor to lay hands on me, I would experience instantaneous healing. Pretty cool, right? Sounds like it anyway. These people remind me of Job's three friends in the Bible. For those of you that have never heard the story, here it is. Through no fault of his own, Job's health was taken away by Satan. His misery was so great that he sat outside under a tree. He was suffering so much that for days he wouldn't eat anything or talk to anyone. Then these three friends came to see him. Poor Job thought they were there to help pick up his spirit and give him encouragement. Instead, they criticized him and insulted him. Boy, no wonder the saying "With friends like these, who needs enemies?" came about.

Jobanites—that's what I personally call these people. Nope, they are not anything like Job. But they sure act like his friends. Over the years,

I've noticed that when the going gets tough for someone, these Jobanites suddenly seem to appear out of nowhere. And for all their much talking, they do nothing but discourage, confuse, and disillusion people.

If healing was exactly what they claim it should be like, then all that remains is for all that multitude of church ministers with the gift of healing to go out like Jesus did during his time and begin healing all the sick. If they would stick to their word concerning healing, they would travel from city to city and practically empty our hospitals of sick folk. Not only won't they do it, but the fact is they can't do it. Ironically enough, right after condemning my cancer because of my own supposed weak faith and unbelief, their pastor's spouse died from an illness. And a short time later, the pastor wound up in the hospital from health complications too.

My wife endured a lot of pressure and spiritual accusations from her friend but not once rebuked her for it. Time itself took care of that. My friend, God is not mocked. The glory and honor for healing belongs to him and him alone.

As you probably guessed it by now, we never did drive over to our friend's church. Do you think we were foolish in not doing so? We don't think so. And I am fixing to show you why.

I am going to give you six examples here. They are nothing short of being pure gold nuggets from the Word of God concerning healing. Just read on and enjoy them. And don't forget that the Bible does tell us in 2 Timothy 2:15, "Study to shew thyself approved unto God, a workman that needeth not to be ashamed, rightly dividing the word of truth."

Chapter 10

GOLD NUGGETS FROM THE BIBLE

1. 2 Timothy 4:20—The apostle Paul takes off from Miletus, leaving Trophimus behind sick. Couldn't the great apostle Paul have healed him before leaving? Sure he could. But why didn't he?

2. 2 Kings 20:6—The king Hezekiah was destined to die in bed from an illness. But God answered his prayer for healing and promised to add into him another fifteen years of life. Although healing is promised in verse 6, we see later in verse 7 the prophet Isaiah doctoring Hezekiah, using a home remedy made out of figs. Why was he doing that if the promise had already been made?

3. John 11:6—Lazarus, a close friend of Jesus and a true believer in God, died without ever getting his prayer for healing answered

4. Acts 9:36—In the city of Joppa, a believer named Tabitha, who was called Dorcas, became so sick that she died. I know of one sure thing, and that is that Christians always pray for one another. Do you not think that they prayed for her? Then why did she die?

5. Jeremiah 42:4—The prophet Jeremiah prayed to God on behalf of the people. Of course, he could use an answer right then and

there, but God didn't answer him until ten days later. Let me ask you this: what if God, instead of ten days, had answered after ten years? How about thirty-eight years?

6. John 5:5—This man had an infirmity for thirty-eight years but could never get healed. Why? Surely not because of his lack of faith. He was a strong believer. No, rather it was because he was too slow in trying to get himself into the pool where the angel stood.

I am willing to bet that if these Jobanites had lived at the time of these people's lives, they would've pointed their bony finger at them and accuse them of having their prayers go unanswered because of unbelief. Friend, remember that the Lord doesn't jump to our rescue every single time that we call upon him. Some people must think they can use him like a light switch or something. The one and true answer for all this is this—and this is not my opinion either, but it's what the Word of God actually teaches—when one prays for anything, whether it's for health, marriage, finances, etc., no matter what in the world the petition is for, God's answer will always be

1. NO, never
2. YES, right now, immediately
3. YES, but wait until later

Sometimes it's so much later that one tends to get discouraged. Don't let that happen to you. If anything, the Lord is always on time on everything. Yes, even when the answer is no. Because if it's no, then it's for your own good. You might come back at me with "You mean the answer to my prayer might be no, and I could die."

Let me ask you this. Do you mean to tell me that with everything you've ever read and heard about heaven, you wouldn't want to go there?

And if you did go there, you would want to come back here? No way. I can't believe that. Let me show you something to think about. If death is that bad, then why does God say in the Bible, "Precious in the sight of the Lord is the death of his saints."

August 1—Saturday morning, Beatrice, accompanied by April, drove me to the Methodist Hospital, where I was quickly checked in. Prior arrangements had been made for us by our oncologist back in Corpus Christi. We finally met with Dr. Bachier, medical specialist in hematology and oncology. His subspecialty is blood and marrow transplant. Joe, whom he kiddingly claimed was his right-hand man, we didn't meet until later. He jokingly said he'd never get anything done if it wasn't for Joe's help. Well, wouldn't you know it. Joe turned out to be *Jo*.

We were all surprised when she walked into our waiting room and introduced herself as Jo, a registered nurse. She also happened to be the transplant coordinator. She laughed when we told her that we had been expecting Joe the man to show up. These two, along with the rest of the medical staff, always managed to keep me on my toes. Just like the staff back in Corpus Christi, their personal concern and kindness they showed us really touched our hearts. Every single one of them had a great attitude about them. And their sense of humor was pretty good too. Once again, we were sure that the Lord had brought us here for a very special purpose. And that was not just for healing but also to show us that in the midst of our misery and suffering, God is also there with us, showing his love and concern for us through those that love him.

Later during the day, our little family took a walk throughout the whole floor where I would be staying. We had never seen so many people sick with cancer before. Some had their bodies completely decimated by the cancer. Others seemed to look okay. I already knew what I looked like. I wondered what Kind of Impression I was making on the visitors. I knew one thing for sure. Death had us on its clutches, and most people don't like to see that on anyone, especially those that are close to them.

August 19—Today I received what was known as an autologous bone marrow transplant. About a week back, a long straw-type needle was inserted on the right side of the base of my neck. It went inside one of my main arteries near my heart. At the end of it, which barely stuck out in front of my neck, was attached what seemed to be one piece of surgical tubing approximately three to four inches in length. Through these my blood would be taken out of my body. The blood would travel through some medical equipment and return back into my body. But not before the necessary bone marrow cell were taken out of it. They were going to deep-freeze them, and after everything was over, they would return them back into my body. Hopefully, that would be the last medical episode that I would go through.

During this month, I also got to receive the much talked about harsh chemo everyone had been talking about. Back in Corpus Christi, they had said that this would be the real McCoy of them all. They weren't kidding. Since it had been two whole months with no chemo, my hair had already begun to spring up all over my head. Everybody was used to seeing me with a bald, shiny head. Now they would marvel when they would see me come over with a new crop of hair. Even Beatrice was proud of me now. She had begun calling me her fuzzy head. Well, it didn't take very long. I quickly lost it all again.

As I found out later, losing my hair was the least of my troubles. My memory got worse. The devil's door on my life had been opened once more. Fever, nausea, headaches, and everything else one could think of, I began going through all over again. Throughout the duration of this disease we documented at least 42 side effects plus well over 100 different types of medications. that I endured. I felt like I was in a daze the whole time.

By this time, our daughter had already left to go back to Lawrence, Kansas. She had returned to make classroom preparation for the new school year. This meant Beatrice had her hands full with me now. Some days I spent in the RV. Others, I spent in the hospital. More in the hospital, though. Jo had given my wife an important job that had to be done at home for me. She had been given a large folder and told to write down on it all the different types of medications I would be taking and my different reactions to each one of them. On the days that we did get to spend in the RV, I still had to be driven back and forth to the hospital for my Neupogen injections once in the morning. Later, I began going morning and night too.

It got so bad for me that I soon began hallucinating. My brain was really fried now, I thought. It started one night when we were sleeping in our little RV. I didn't know if I just woke up or was already awake. I do recall looking out my window by the bunk bed and seeing a group of people there. Some were sitting around a table. Others were standing. They were talking about something. Then several of them looked over to where I was and started asking me to come on over to where they were. The next instant, I was standing by the door ready to go outside. I don't even remember how I got to the door, but there I was. I then began arguing with Beatrice. I insisted on leaving, arguing with her that people were calling me outside. She at last managed to restrain me and keep me from leaving. These were strange episodes, but she was able to manage anyhow.

I remember waking up in the middle of the night and just sitting there in a drugged-out stupor. Beatrice had just gotten up either to go to the restroom or to get a drink of water. I couldn't tell which. She started speaking to me, but I couldn't understand a word of what she was telling me. You see, ever since I had sat up in bed, I had been hearing these real ugly, horrible noises inside my head. Everything I heard would vibrate and echo while at the same time making a terrible noise. I figured right then and there that these horrible noises I was hearing must certainly be sounds one would hear in hell itself. This had happened to me while I was in Portland, but here in San Antonio, it had gotten a lot worse. At first when this had begun to happen, it had rocked my little world. But with much prayer, I had finally learned to accept it and live with it. I mean, what choice did I have? I just prayed that his grace would be all sufficient for me and that I would not give up my faith in him.

The fevers were okay too. At a steady 99°F to 101°F, they were all right. We could live with that. Eventually, one did manage to get out of hand. Once again I found myself being driven to the hospital at one thirty in the morning and straight into ICU. Man, I could've died that night because of a high fever. But the medication, documentation, and monitoring Beatrice had been doing on me finally had paid off. Boy, what a great blessing it is to be loved by a beautiful and wonderful Christian wife like her. I thank God for giving her to me as a lifelong partner and will continue to do so all the days of my life.

Chapter 12

MORE TRIALS AND ERRORS

During my trials there at Methodist Hospital, Pastor Lee Patton and his wonderful wife, Irene, proved to be the just the type of encouragement that I needed at the time. Brother Lee had gone through stage 4 lymphoma, and he had made it. He was a survivor and knew exactly what we were going through. During that month, they invited us to dinner and received us into their home like regular family. Even though I couldn't taste the food, I sure enjoyed the fellowship. Isn't God good? Yes, all the time.

When I came out of ICU for the second time, I felt like all my insides had dried up. My felt so dry and parched that it had become very painful to swallow. Even water hurt going down my throat. Soon I was put on a liquid diet. Swallowing food was out of the question. I had tried that, and when the food was going down my intestines, it felt like someone was cutting up my insides. It made me feel like my chest and stomach were being ripped from the inside.

One day while I was in my usual daze, I suddenly came to my senses and found myself crawling in the middle of the corridor of the hospital. I didn't know how I got there. All I knew was that I was sick as a dog and was throwing up all over the place. Beatrice and several nurses were trying their best to pick me off the floor, but they couldn't. It felt to me like I had just waken up from a bad dream. I felt so embarrassed by the whole thing afterward. Not to mention all the trouble I was causing the poor nurses on that floor.

I do recall one day when I almost scared a nurse completely out of her shoes. It wasn't intentional, though. Here's what happened. During one of the times that I was hooked up for the bone marrow transplant, I just lay there being a good patient for once when one of the hoses that were attached to my neck came loose all by itself. Next thing I knew, there was blood flying all over the place. At that particular time, Beatrice had left the room where the marrow transplant took place. And only the nurse and I were there. There was no one else there, but the curtain had still been drawn to ensure me even more privacy.

The dumb surgical tubing had gone completely wild, whiplashing blood all over my small enclosure where only moments ago I had felt safe and secure. At last I managed to grab the tubing and pinch off the end. Slippery as it was, I don't know how I did it, but I held on to it anyway. Doing this, I quickly yelled out to the nurse. All I remember then was that the curtain was a blur as it was thrown back suddenly and there was a wild scream of panic. My wife and others just happened to walk into the room when all this took place. Next thing I knew, there was chaos in the room. I was covered almost completely in blood. My bald head was shiny red now. But not everything went bad in the hospital. Sometimes good things happened too.

August 29th—It was evening already, and I had been feeling a little sad all day. It was my wife's birthday, and here I was stuck in the hospital with health so bad that I was unable to take her anywhere. We were talking quietly when in walked Fernando and Nydia. They are both brethren in the Lord and work in the San Antonio area. Fernando is a constable, and Nydia is a schoolteacher. Fernando also went through a battle against cancer and is still here with us because of God's wonderful grace. We had fellowship together, and they encouraged us. Then they prayed for us and gave us a loving hug. But just before they left, they said God had impressed it in their hearts to give us a blessing. Saying this, they placed over $200 into Beatrice's hand and told her it was for her birthday.

Yes, that August of 2009 could well be said to have been not only a very interesting month in my life but also a very wonderful one too. For a while there, I almost became a statistic, but by God's grace, I was able to miraculously survive. Marty and Lynn Israel, our brethren in the Lord, say I am a survivor. Well, if I am, it's by the Lord's good will and not my own. I can personally vouch for that tidbit of info.

I was criticized many times for my happy, cheerful attitude. Those closest to me said that I practically had both feet in the grave and that I wouldn't last even six months. Cold and callous, wouldn't you say so? To this, I can only reply with the scripture in the Bible that says, "Great peace have they which love thy law: and nothing shall offend them" (Psalm 119:165).

I remember one day when Beatrice and I visited the Sunday school class at First Baptist for the first time. When they found out who I was, they exclaimed in surprise, "So you're the one we've been praying for." They then started hugging me, shaking my hand, and patting me in the back, telling how happy they were to see me doing so well. They told me that they had been praying for me for a year. I was so shocked to hear that. I shouldn't have been, but I was.

What had happened was that my wife's boss, Larry Curtis, had found out through her that I had cancer. So immediately he had informed his Sunday school class about it. I had been in their prayer list ever since. I recall how surprise everyone had been when they found out who I was. To them it was a great testimony of how the Lord answers prayer. To me and Beatrice, it showed us just a little bit of what heaven is going to be like.

September 2—I was finally released to go home. The devil had hurt me, pounded me, and assaulted me in every way possible. But thanks to the Lord that, like Job, he enabled me not to give up but to continue to have faith on him. I know that many people under heavy persecution or great physical turmoil do give up on God and give up the will to live. Eventually, they die. And that's very sad and so unnecessary. A Christian will not die until God calls that brother or sister home. No matter how critically ill they are or how bad they look health-wise, they cannot leave this world until the Lord allows it.

Chapter 13

GOD'S SPIRITUAL ARMOR

November 16—Today, I made a barbecue. Beatrice had just arrived from work. We greeted each other with a hug and a kiss as we have always done and then sat down and talked. After we talked for a few minutes, she got up and went into the house. As I sat there alone and watched the fire going, my mind began to wander. I thought of that dream I had experienced one night almost a year ago, a terrible dream where I had fought long and hard against Satan, and of how disappointed I had been at my own inability to defeat him.

Looking back, I fully understand the meaning of that dream. In that fight, I never really had to win. You see, the battle had already been won for me. For all of us as a matter of fact. Our Lord Jesus fought him and defeated him by allowing himself to be nailed to a cruel cross at the place of the skull, called Calvary. In the dream, the Lord gave me the necessary strength to withstand Satan's attack. And no matter what he threw at me or dished out, I was able to withstand. Because I was wearing the full armor of God, he was never able to knock me down.

In the book of Ephesians chapter 6, verse 11, we are commanded by God—not asked, but commanded—to put on the whole armor that we might be able to stand against Satan's wiles. In the old days, Roman soldiers would've never marched into battle without having put on their full battle gear. To neglect their shield or some other piece of their protective equipment would've been foolish on their part. Likewise, you and I should use wisdom in fighting spiritual battles. And we would do well to remember that the battle is the Lord's and not ours alone.

Should healing come to you, never forget of whom you received it from. Whatever prayer has been answered for you, be sure to give God the glory for it. Wherever you go, give testimony of what great things the Lord has done for you in your life. Like Pastor Sutton preached in church once, there are two things that concern us when it comes to "the choice to rejoice." And they are these, "Rejoice is either for the taking or the making."

My whole story can be summed up by these two scriptures: "Be careful for nothing; but in everything by prayer and supplication with thanksgiving let your requests be made known unto God. And the peace of God, which passeth all understanding, shall keep your hearts and minds through Christ Jesus" (Philippians 4:6-7).

December 20th—While my lovely wife and I were in church worshipping the Lord, I received a text message on my cell from the PET Scan Center in Corpus Christi. This is what it said: "Your PET scan results just came in, and we are pleased to inform you that you are now cancer-free."

Sabino lives with his lovely wife, Beatrice, in Portland, Texas. He is a welder by trade, and his wife is an employee of the Portland Independent School District. After his encounter with lymphoma, she now calls him her boy. He calls her Bea, which means "beautiful" in Spanish. Both are now faithful members at the First Baptist Church in Portland under the pastoralship of Dr. Robert E. Sutton Jr.